PCOS DIET BOOK: A COLLECTION OF RECIPES TO BEAT THE SYMPTOMS OF PCOS

A Cookbook For Women Suffering From PCOS

By: Chantelle Williams

TABLE OF CONTENTS

Publishers Notes

Disclaimer

This publication is intended to provide helpful and informative material. It is not intended to diagnose, treat, cure, or prevent any health problem or condition, nor is intended to replace the advice of a physician. No action should be taken solely on the contents of this book. Always consult your physician or qualified health-care professional on any matters regarding your health and before adopting any suggestions in this book or drawing inferences from it.

The author and publisher specifically disclaim all responsibility for any liability, loss or risk, personal or otherwise, which is incurred as a consequence, directly or indirectly, from the use or application of any contents of this book.

Any and all product names referenced within this book are the trademarks of their respective owners. None of these owners have sponsored, authorized, endorsed, or approved this book.

Always read all information provided by the manufacturers' product labels before using their products. The author and publisher are not responsible for claims made by manufacturers.

Kindle Edition 2012

Worldwide Copyright 2012

Magnum Results Corp.

British Columbia, Canada

DEDICATION

I want to dedicate this book to Andrea Snowden who has been a tremendous help to me while getting over issues with my health and eventually having the child that made my life complete.

CHAPTER 1- LET'S LOOK INTO PCOS

PCOS is the acronym for Polycystic Ovarian Syndrome. It is a disorder of the hormones that affects roughly 7% of all women. It is a known fact that this hormonal disorder is specific to women.

According to professionals, the actual amount of affected women with this disease might reach a high number of 1 out of every 10; the reason is simply because a lot of cases are not undiagnosed. The question is usually asked why there are so many cases of undiagnosed polycystic ovarian syndrome. Since the symptoms can differ from one woman to the next it is frequently difficult to correctly diagnose if the woman is experiencing polycystic ovarian syndrome.

Most women have never heard of PCOS; but it causes a large variety of symptoms that frequently affect the reproductive health of females in ways that have the potential of being really devastating. Though PCOS frequently affects the females' reproductive system, there is importance in understanding that this is a disorder of the endocrine system.

Often polycystic ovarian syndrome causes long-term significant health consequences, therefore; it is good to get an accurate and quick diagnosis, which should be followed by the proper course of treatment.

PCOS can be characterized by ovaries that have been enlarged, and have numerous painless and small cysts. Indications of the disorder polycystic ovarian syndrome are: lipid abnormalities, obesity, acne, male-patterned thinning hair, absent or irregular periods, infertility, having excess growth of hair on your body and/or face.

Where individuals are experiencing two of these symptoms or more, it is recommended they visit a physician, favorably a reproductive endocrinologist.

Can a genetic connection be found in females who experience the disorder?

Though the vulnerability to PCOs is frequently inherited, the precise cause is unidentified. Most frequently, PCOS symptoms start with the beginning of the menstrual cycle; however, the symptoms can be experienced earlier during the preteen years or could develop at any period throughout the period when she can bear children.

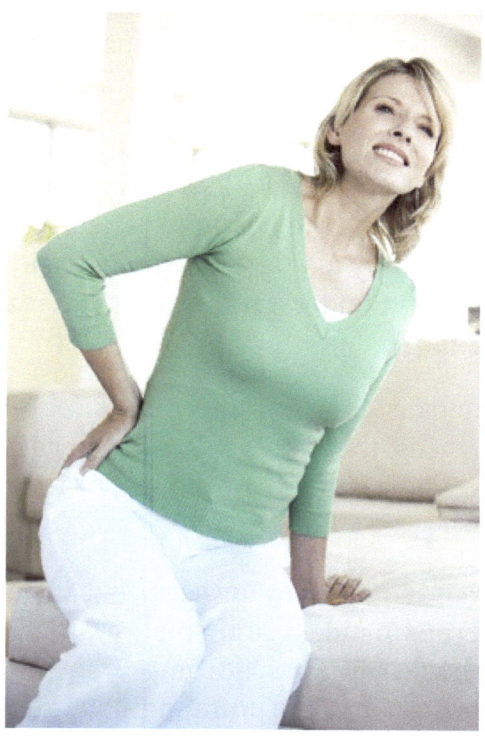

As women get older the polycystic ovarian syndrome becomes less common and it is particularly uncommon among women who are post-menopausal. Unfortunately there are consequences of the condition, like lipid abnormalities and diabetes, occurring for a long time after menopause.

It is a disorder of hormones... What exactly are hormones?

Steroids or proteins that are directly secreted in your blood stream are known as hormones. A lot of the body's every day, normal functions are controlled hormonal substances like pregnancy, reproduction, sexual function, persons' responses to stress, regulations of fluids and metabolism of minerals. Glands like that of ovaries, medulla and adrenal cortex, pancreas, parathyroid, thyroid, hypothalamus and pituitary are what make up your endocrine system which have the responsibility of producing hormones in females. When there are malfunctions or breakdowns during the hormonal process, the body is significantly affected.

How can PCOS be diagnosed?

A lot of doctors make a diagnosis for polycystic ovarian syndrome centered on the abovementioned symptoms; however, confirming a diagnosis needs more than basic acknowledgment of these symptoms. To confirm polycystic ovarian syndrome, blood testing is required for a range of hormones. The production of these hormones is by the thyroid gland, pituitary gland, adrenal glands plus the ovaries.

A complete assessment of PCOS includes a complete physical examination plus laboratory testing for insulin, glucose, triglyceride and cholesterol. Keep in mind that the most qualified doctor is a reproductive endocrinologist and he or she can diagnose plus treat PCOS accurately.

What available treatments exist for females with polycystic ovary syndrome?

Largely, the PCOS treatment is dependent on the experience of the symptoms of each individual female, as well as whether or not she has fertility issues. If the woman is not interested in having a baby, oral contraceptives are effectual in regulating the menstrual cycles, decreasing the level of male hormones, plus reducing your risk of getting uterine cancer.

There are treatments for the signs of polycystic ovary syndrome. These comprise of: Surgical therapy, Fertility therapy using ovulation-inducing drugs, GnRH analogs, Anti-androgens, sensitizing insulin- anti-diabetes drugs, oral contraceptives, synthetic progesterone's (Progestin's) and weight loss if you are obese or overweight.

Frequently Polycystic ovarian syndrome is related to a variety of serious medical illnesses. These conditions include sensitivity to insulin reduction, which could lead to individuals increasing their risk of getting cardiovascular disease and diabetes mellitus. Also, PCOS could be related to uterine cancer.

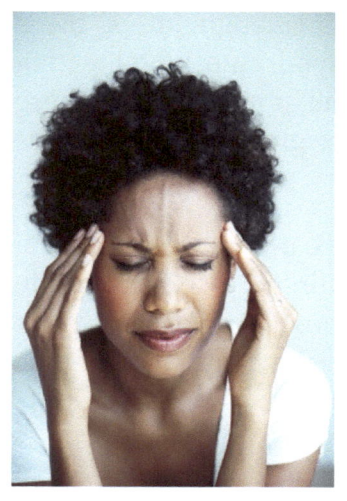

There are many women, who experience PCOS symptoms that trigger emotional concerns like depression. These symptoms can be very distressing because they cause the growth of body and facial hair, obesity and infertility. Females having polycystic ovary syndrome require social and emotional support to constructively handle the consequences that this disorder might place on their lives.

Can I be of any help?

If you know someone who has been diagnosed with this hormonal disorder, you can help by being there to offer support through their challenges and listen to them vent. This gives them confront as they struggle to win this battle for a satisfying, healthy lifestyle. It has been shown in research that a sturdy network of family and friends is an incredible asset to females with PCOS, as the support system enhances their capability of coping with the syndrome effects.

Although the causes of PCOS remain unidentified and there is really no cure, awareness in the public can contribute a great much to help females learn to identify the symptoms so they can obtain an exact diagnosis.

There is no secret in the fact that weight gain and PCOS is connected. Within the United States there is an increasing awareness of the crisis of obesity. This has resulted in a flood of diet programs that assures dramatic results. However, many of these offer none or little scientific data for the backing of these claims, while another great number are hard to maintain.

Frequently, most persons return to their original eating habits after a period of time, typically after they have lost the weight, then they regain it and sometimes more. This is particularly true of females diagnosed with PCOS. Since weight loss and dieting is so hard, it is common for females to try many varieties of diet programs; then they wonder if a PCOS diet is available that will work.

Many ponder if a diet low in carbohydrate is suitable for a woman having PCOS since there is an insulin resistance link. In fact, a diet low in carbohydrates has not been proven effective in long-term successes in weight loss related to PCOS. Additionally, the high quantities of fat and protein and regularly saturated fats are known to be dangerous when consumed in large amounts over an extended period of time. Participating in such diets can increase your risk further for high cholesterol, high blood pressure and heart disease.

However, diets low in fat are frequently unproductive as well. Individuals who follow this kind of diet often consume many foods rich in carbohydrates. Basic refined carbohydrates such as white sugar, pasta, potatoes and rice can rapidly elevate the levels of insulin. Extended periods with high insulin could eventually result in insulin resistance. As such, this can prolong the PCOS cycle of symptoms, weight gain, and insulin resistance as well as androgen levels.

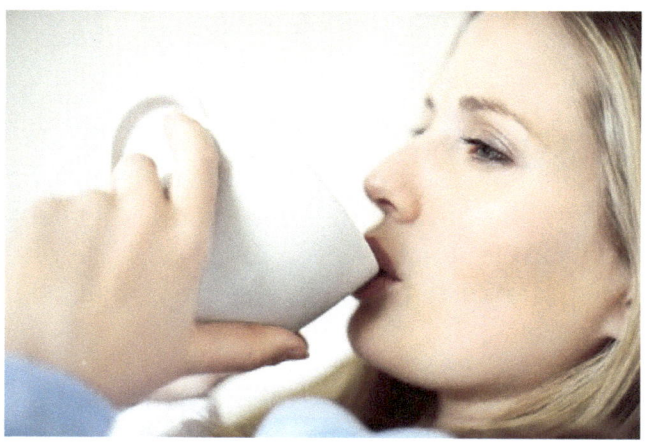

Regular exercise and good nutrition are the secrets to experiencing long-term, steady results. Even though weight loss might not be as much as desired, eating foods that are healthy and remaining active are top-notch methods of maintaining good health.

Certainly it is beneficial if persons cut back on white or simple carbohydrates such as pasta, potatoes, rice and white sugar. However, putting in additional carbohydrates and complex grains do contribute to several important health benefits such as antioxidants and fiber.

TIP 1 Stop deficiency dieting

Do you know the real meaning of the word "diet"? The true meaning of diet is nutrition or nourishment. This implies wellness and health, not deprivation.

What does the word 'diet' mean to you? The real definition of 'diet' means nourishment or nutrition. This implies health and wellness—not starvation. Nevertheless there are so many famous diets today that are associated with distress and pain. Persons fail to realize that healthy eating should and can be enjoyable.

Stop by a health food store nearby for information on how to add natural delicious foods like vegetables, lentils and organic, local ingredients to your everyday meals. Several health food stores provide take-home and deli food supplies that could make your food preparation for PCOS easier.

American Diabetes Association is also able to provide you with healthy recipes for PCOS.

Tip 2 Blood sugar control

PCOS weight gain can be linked to irregularities in glucose and insulin metabolism. Insulin's primary job is controlling your blood sugar. However, insulin also tells your body to store fat. Insulin in high levels increases the production of androgens, which could worsen symptoms of PCOS.

With (IR) insulin resistance, the blood sugar levels will increase despite the high levels of insulin and Type 2 diabetes might eventually result. With positive diet changes and exercise, this might delay the onset of diabetes. A PCOS diet reduces the quantity of sugary carbs you may eat and offers you

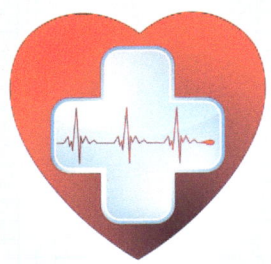

weight-loss benefits.

To make healthy changes in the PCOS diet, cut out snack foods, some fruits, cereals, potatoes, pasta and white breads. Replace those foods with PCOS diet-healthy options such as the following: Foods having healthy fats (fish, nuts, and olive oil), foods rich in protein (legumes, lean meats), high-fiber carbs, and nutrient dense.

Ask your registered dietitian or a doctor for a list of foods to try, and another with a list of foods to avoid. Practice eating mini-meals during the day -- this will keep your levels of blood sugar even.

TIP 3 Daily Exercises

It is obvious that exercise is technically not a 'nutritious' diet tip; however, if you are seeking to burn calories, every day exercise is a must. First make a visit to your doctor, and as soon as you get permission to go-ahead, start moving. A perfect complement to any PCOS diet is exercise, especially for women with type 2 diabetes, insulin resistance or PCOS. Regular exercise is necessary and wonderful for each of us, and below are few reasons why.

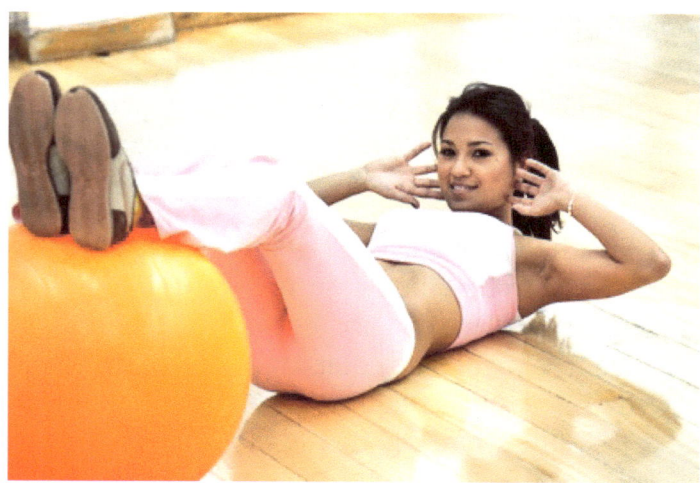

Exercise: weight loss is increased; for pregnancy it gets women in top shape physically; increases your body's natural opioids (endorphins); provides a mood boost; blood glucose levels is regulated. Being physically fit also might help you in carrying a healthy bouncing baby to full term and have a delivery that is uncomplicated.

Tip 4 Evaluate your food relationship

If you are passionate about eating and desire success in a PCOS diet, one must rethink their relationship with food. Some women reward themselves with food for accomplishing something or as an emotional solace if feeling blue or lonely. Others get excited about their next meal sitting in a favorite restaurant or prepare food as means of bringing friends and family together.

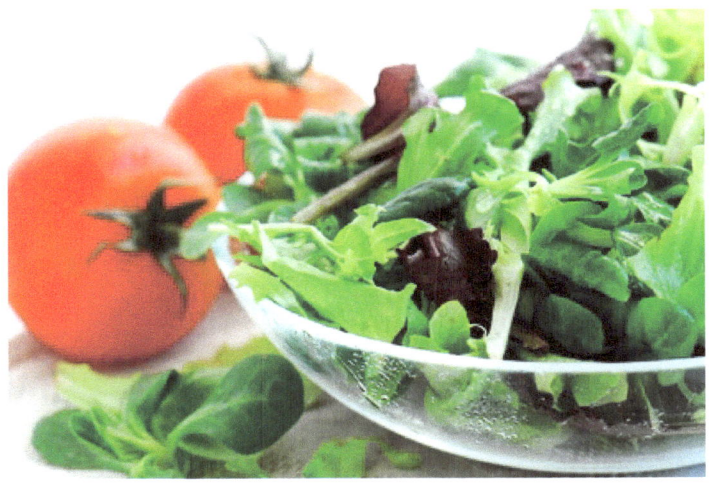

A secret behind PCOS diet is reframing your thoughts where you eat to live not live to eat. Select foods that are nutrient dense and filling. Instead of comfort food, junk food or party foods that will only add more pounds and fat, eat foods that will add nourishment to your body. However, it is perfectly acceptable for you to occasionally enjoy rich, delicious foods -- but in moderation only. If you find yourself having an unhealthy food relationship, like starving yourself, purging, binging ... help is available.

TIP 5 Ask about metformin

Glucophage (Metformin) is a developed drug for type 2 diabetes and frequently is (off label) prescribed for PCOS and obesity. Metformin might offer help to women pursuing a PCOS diet. Benefits include: fertility drugs sensitivity is improved; restoring normal periods; levels of androgens is decreased; improving cholesterol levels; lowering blood pressure; helps with loss of weight.

Remember, PCOS is no one's fault. However, it is in the individual's hands to collaborate with their doctor to find solutions for PCOS diet and learn how to live with this common hormonal problem in the healthiest way possible.

Chapter 2 - Low Glycemic Index (GI) Recipes For PCOS – Quick, Easy And Delicious

Apricot Compote with Tuna Steak

The oils discovered in fish-like tuna are loaded with omega-3, a 'good fat' believed to help preserve a wholesome heart. The recipe that follows combines savory low GI (Glycemic Index) compote made from apricots and tomatoes with tuna. GI is a measure of how quickly blood sugar levels (e.g. levels of glucose in the blood) rise after eating various foods – and how it may affect a woman with PCOS.

Ingredients

(Per person)

1 tuna steak (about 150g)

1 tomato, medium

1 tbsp brandy

½ half small red onion

8 apricots, dried

½ teaspoon of dried thyme

Freshly ground pepper

1 tbsp balsamic vinegar

2 tbsp extra virgin olive oil

Crisp lettuce leaves (a few)

Chop finely -- half the tomato and half the dried apricots, then put into a blender with the thyme, olive oil, vinegar, brandy, and a large helping of pepper. Next blend together the ingredients and marinate the tuna in the sauce for thirty minutes; best if done at room temperature. When marinating for longer, store the tuna in a refrigerator until 30 minutes prior to preparing.

As soon as the tuna is marinated sufficiently, slice the onion in strips then fry lightly for two minutes. The tomato remaining should be sliced and fried along with the rest of the apricot for an additional minute. Layer the onions and arrange the tomatoes and apricots on washed lettuce.

Use a spatula to remove the fish from marinade and fry the marinade and tuna in the same pot. If you prefer the steak to be slightly rare in the middle the steak should be strictly cooked for two minutes on both sides. Be cautioned that this method for cooking does not guarantee the bacteria inside the fish will be killed. If this is a concern then cook for three minutes on both sides.

Lentil Cakes & Roasted Mushroom

These lentil cakes and mushrooms are as tasty as they are healthy, and contain low GI and fat, plus provide a great source for vegetarians.

Suggested Nutritional Information

(Per serving): Fiber: 11g, 522mg of Sodium, Fat: 12g (Cholesterol: 0mg, Saturated: 1g) Calories: 251, Sugars: 5g, Carbohydrate: 26g, Protein: 11g

Ingredients

(Serves 4)

½ cup/100g red dried lentils

2 cups/150g crimini mushrooms/chestnut mushrooms, sliced

75g /2/3 cup walnuts, chopped

An egg

1 onion, medium

2 tsp soy sauce

1 tbsp Worcestershire sauce

1 teaspoon Italian seasoning /mixed herbs

For 10 minutes in boiling water cook the lentils then skim off all scum; let simmer for an additional 15 minutes. Meanwhile chop the onion, walnuts and mushrooms very finely.

The lentils should be drained, and when cooled mix with all other ingredients in a mixing bowl. Use your hands to mix the ingredients together.

Using a little butter, lightly grease the baking tray. Form the mixture in 4 equally sized cakes utilizing a cutter for pastry or similar then put them on the baking greased tray. Next, cook at Gas Mark 5 /380°F /190°C for twenty-five to thirty minutes. Then roast some cherry tomatoes, carrots and sweet potatoes, and serve simultaneously with the sugar snap peas and cakes. Particularly, they are good if served with some vegetable gravy.

Parsley and Lemon Chicken

These parcels of chicken have a great tangy taste them plus they make a healthy meal that can be had anytime throughout the year.

Ingredients

(Should serve 3)

3 med chicken breasts

½ melon lemon

A handful of garden-fresh parsley

3 cocktail sticks

Freshly ground pepper

½ teaspoon salt

1 tablespoon olive oil

3 garlic cloves

The lemon peel should be removed and dice into small pieces. The garlic should be finely sliced then chop the parsley and mix in a bowl with the lemon. In another bowl mix pepper and salt.

Carefully slice all the chicken breasts (in lengths) to create a little pocket. Avoid slicing right through so the pocket is able to be sealed as soon as the lemon is placed in it.

Put a large helping of your lemon mixture in all the breasts then using a cocktail stick seal the pocket.

Put the breasts in a dish that is oven proof, use foil to cover then cook for thirty minutes at Gas Mark 5/380°F/190°C. After remove the foil then cook for another 5 minutes, this will allow your breasts to brown. It can be served with a fresh salad.

Dill Salmon Grilled with Olive Sauce

Salmon is not only a low GI food but also it is a source high in omega-3. This is a good fat rich in anti-oxidants. Where there is concern regarding the mercury deposits found in salmon, you can consider eating only wild salmon, even though it is a little more pricey.

Suggested Nutritional Information per serving

938mg of Sodium, 2g of Fiber, 13g of Carbohydrate (7g of Sugars) 13g of Fat (Cholesterol: 75mg, Saturated: 3g), 32g of Protein, 299of Calories

Ingredients

(Serves 3)

3 salmon fillets (medium sized)

1 lemon

2 teaspoons dried dill or chopped fresh

200g /One cup olives black olives

Fresh parsley (a handful)

300g /1¼ cups natural yogurt

Salt (One pinch)

Line a suitable tray that can fit under the grill then put the salmon fillets in it. Next cut the lemon then squeeze ½ of the juice on the salmon and sprinkle with ½ the dill. For four minutes cook under a medium grill then remove. Flip over then coat the next section of the salmon using the remaining dill and lemon juice. Cook by placing it under the grill for another four minutes.

While cooking the salmon, chop the parsley and the olives into little pieces. Mix together the parsley and olives with the yogurt with salt (a pinch) and serve as the complement to the salmon.

Chocolate Vegetarian Chili

Vegetarian chili is a recipe that has been spiced using a Mexican style with the adding of cocoa power into the mixture. Though many persons find this combination interesting, a unique richness is added to the sauce.

Per serving suggested nutritional information:

205 for Calories, 10g of Protein, 1g of Fat (Cholesterol: 0mg, Saturated: 0g), 368mg of Sodium, 13g of Fiber, 44g of Carbohydrate (Sugars: 6g).

Ingredients

(Serves four)

400g /14oz canned kidney beans & 200g /7oz /1 cup green beans

8 cup mushrooms OR 15 mushrooms, button

200g/7oz /1¼ cups sweet corn

1 chili (for taste)

400g /14oz canned tomatoes & 4 tablespoons puree tomato

Balsamic vinegar (1½ tablespoon)

Two cloves garlic

A handful of garden fresh herbs OR two teaspoons mixed dry herbs

Cocoa powder (1½ tablespoons)

Chop the chili in little pieces then mix together using the crushed garlic, cocoa powder, herbs, balsamic vinegar, tomato puree and tomatoes. Use a blender or a hand mixer to prepare a thick sauce.

Chop the green beans in half then lightly fry them with the sliced onions in olive oil. Add the sweet corn, kidney beans and mushrooms, and then fry for a couple minutes longer. Chestnut mushrooms quarters can also be used if button mushrooms is not available.

Add the sauce to the pan, place on a lid then on low heat let it simmer for ten to fifteen minutes.

Nut and Banana Cookies

These succulent and soft cookies have a uniformity that is half way between cookies and cake. The banana adds to each cookie a fruity and moist flavor. Soya/soy flour provides a healthy goodness hidden in every cookie.   Soya/soya flour is available at health food stores.

Suggested Nutritional Information for each cookie: Sodium:

28mg, Fiber: 3g, 21g of Carbohydrate (Sugars: 7g), Protein: 7g, Calories: 170, Fat: 8g (Cholesterol: 31mg, Saturated: 1g).

Ingredients

(Twelve large cookies)

Ripe bananas (4)

2 eggs

170g/2 cups soya/soy flour

25g/¼ cup cashew nuts

60g/½ cups whole meal flour

30g/¼ cup raisins

3 tablespoons olive oil

Baking powder (½ teaspoon)

In a small bowl mash all four bananas with a fork; next, transfer to a bigger cooking bowl. If you don't want to have a lot to clean up, the bananas can be mashed in the big bowl. However, it will be much harder to do.

Mix the whole meal flour and soy slowly in the bananas making until the mixture gets thick.

To form a paste that is smooth, mix in the olive oil and eggs. Add the raisins and cashew nuts and mix them in gently.

Two baking trays should be lined with baking parchment then grease lightly the surface using a little butter. Utilizing two spoons move six big scoops of the mix on both baking trays. For 15 minutes cook in an oven previously heated to Gas Mark 5/380°F /190°C.

Lemon Sponge Cake

Single slice of sponge cake is a tasty desert or an afternoon snack following a meal low in GI. This version is extremely tasty with a lemony flavor. Overall the GI of this cake is lowered by the use of butter and ground almonds. Despite this fact it still has a high sugar content which means that it must only be enjoyed in moderation.

Suggested Nutritional Information for each slice:

Sodium: 75mg, Fiber: 1g, Protein: 2g, Calories: 118, Fat: 6g (Cholesterol: 9mg, Saturated: 2g), Carbohydrate: 16g (Sugars: 9g).

Ingredients

(Twelve slices)

100g/½ cup superfine sugar/caster sugar

50g/¼ cup butter

100g /¾ cup plain white flour

5 eggs (use only 3 egg yolks)

Salt (1pinch)

50g/½ cup ground almonds

1 lemon

Baking powder (2½ teaspoons)

Beat the sugar and butter together with an electric mixer or a wooden spoon till it is white. Include the five egg whites but keep back three yokes of the egg for.   Egg whites should be whisked with the sugar and butter until all is mixed in. Continuously whisk the mixture; this will add some air and make the cake lighter.

Grate the rind off half the lemon, after cutting, juice the entire lemon then add the salt, baking powder, flour, almonds, rind and lemon juice to the mixture along with the three remaining egg yolks. Use a wooden spoon and mix until there is a smooth paste.

Coat 2 small cake tins using a little butter then dust with a bit of flour. Pour same amount of mixture in each tin. The oven should be pre-heated to Gas Mark 5/380°F/190°C and the cakes baked for 20 minutes. Avoid over cooking by checking them after fifteen minutes. If after checking the cakes have a golden color and make a hollow sound when they are tapped then they can be removed from the oven.

Suggested Serving

The cake could be served like a desert using a small quantity of custard and a few raw blueberries.

GI PCOS DIET TIPS

Practical tips for a low GI diet living

The aim of the GI diet is that for the dieter, it does not seem like a diet -- so persons can sustain it longer. Following are some practical tips for the preparation of low GI meals.

Staples

One problem with diets such as the Atkins diet is the elimination of staples. Meat always tastes a whole lot better with carbs. However, with the low GI diet these sacrifices are not necessary. Linseed breads, high soy and long-grain white rice, potatoes, sweet pasta, are 3 low GI staples persons can eat with every meal.

Whole meal pastas or durum wheat used to make white pasta are excellent for easy, quick meals. They can be mixed with seasoning, herbs, peas, tinned tomatoes and bacon for a meal in minutes.

Typically potatoes must be avoided on this low GI diet. However sweet potatoes are allowed, which is wonderful because they taste so great! They can be roasted for 40 minutes roast in an oven then served along with a low GI sauce made from frozen spinach, tinned tomatoes and heated chickpeas.

Long-grain white rice that needs boiling for fifteen minutes or more is the best selection for low GI diet. Two of the better options are instant rice or basmati. This can be served along with a vegetable stir fry and chicken.

Snacks

The purpose of the low GI diet is to make you feel less hungry, thus reducing the desire to snack. But for the occasions where you might feel hungry in-between meals, here are some things you could nibble: prunes, apricots and dried apples, which are all low GI foods, unsalted nuts (in small quantities only), semi-skimmed milk, reduced sugar chocolate (look out for the fat content), a slice of unfilled plain sponge cake, All-Bran (a single bowl), and banana smoothies are also low in fat.

Chapter 3 - The PCOS Cookbook Shopping Guide

According to experts, your heart disease, obesity and disease risk becomes lower as your GI rating is lowered. All the following GI is 55 or lower, a low glycemic foods rating.

Cereal

For individuals who prefer to enjoy some cereal at breakfast time, within the range of low glycemic options you have 5 to select from. Coming in first is All Bran having fiber with a rate of 38, Muesli follows at 43. Bran Buds has GI 47 whilst oatmeal rating is 52. Your options also include Oat Bran which has a rating of 55.

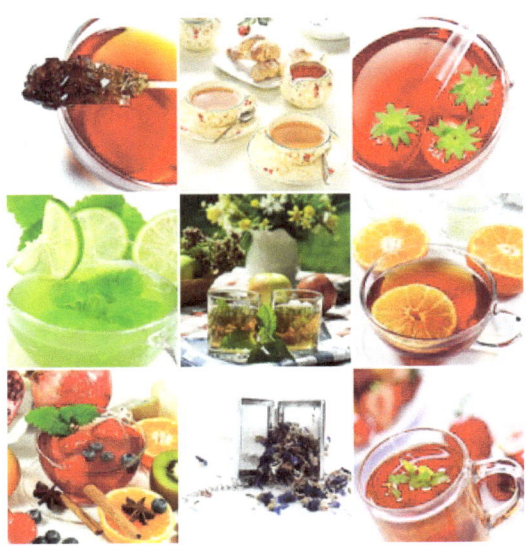

Soup

A hot bowl of steaming soup on a cold winter day always does wonders. There is good news; you still can enjoy a lot of your favorite soup even when on a low GI diet. The lowest ranked is tomato soup at 38; next minestrone is rated at 39. Lentil rounds out the list, with a GI of 44.

Pasta

Yes, pasta can be consumed on any low GI diet. These options are available to you plus they are highly rated. Fettuccini kick things off, it is prepared with egg, and has a 32 rating, next is whole wheat spaghetti having a 37 rating. Star pastina and white spaghetti are tied at a GI of 38, whereas spirals have a 43 rating. Capellini GI ratings are 45, and linguine 46. Finally, there is macaroni with a 47 GI rating.

Vegetables

Five servings are needed every day. However, you must see to it that they fall in the range of low GI. Lettuce, red peppers, onion, mushrooms, cabbage, and broccoli, all have a GI rating of 10. Following is green peas with a 48 GI rating, then carrots at 49.

Fruit

From all the food options, the widest variety comes from fruits. Cherries are first with a rating of 22 GI, next is grapefruit with a rating of 25. Prunes come in third with a 29 rating, whereas dried apricots have a rating of 30. Fresh pears, canned peaches and apples, each have a 38 GI rating and plums have a 39 GI rating. Strawberries come in next having a GI of forty, while fresh peaches and navel oranges are rated 42. Falling in at 43 is canned pears; grapes follow with a 46 DI rating. With a GI rating of 51 you can enjoy mango, plus bananas still can be paired with a bowl of morning oats, they have a 52 GI rating. Finishing off the list is fruit cocktail having a GI of 55.

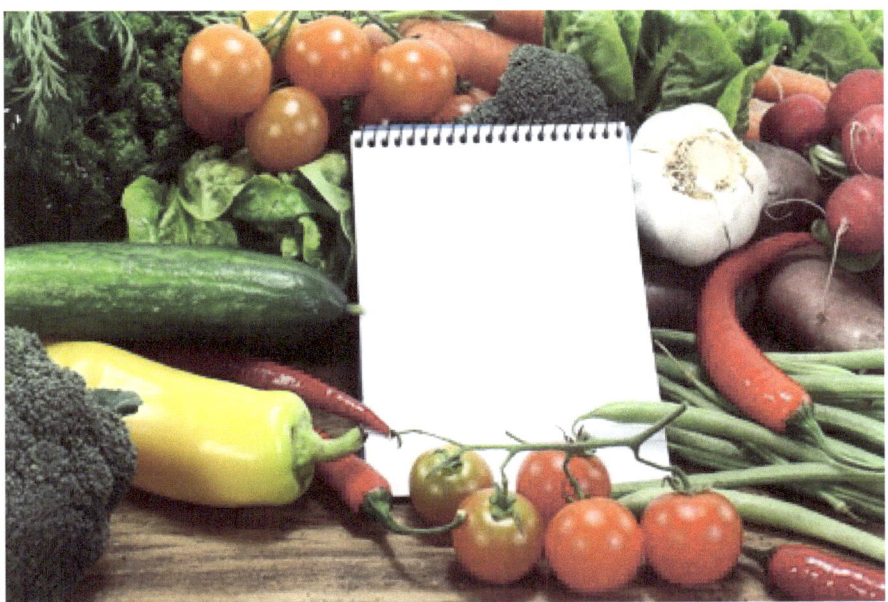

Since the nutrients of low GI foods are slowly absorbed, they will keep the individual feeling full for longer periods of time after they eat. Apart from that persons are more likely to eat less carbs during the day. If you control your blood sugar levels and carb intake with low GI meals, your body can be kept in the best state for weight loss. With stable blood sugar and energy levels, persons can maximize the fat-burning process, aiding persons in reaching their goals faster.

Low GI foods selection

As a basic guide: GI value of seventy or more is a high, GI value of 56-69 is medium, less than 55 is said to be low GI

Below are few top foods with low GI you can include in your diet plan:

Cherries

You might get the feeling that you are spoiling yourself with a sweet treat; however, cherries actually provide you some wonderful diet benefits. It has a GI of 20 (some varieties have a lower GI), which makes cherries a healthy snack for any period of day.

Grapefruit

Having a GI of only 20, they are a wonderful choice. These tangy deliciously fruits have rich levels of micro-nutrients and fiber, so they can be a great breakfast option capable of keeping you feeling satisfied throughout the morning. Perhaps grapefruit really is the most common low GI fruit plus it is frequently considered to be the ideal 'diet food' which is a bit cliché. Some studies show that grapefruit enzymes have fat-burning advantages as well.

They can even be mixed with some strawberries to make a fruit salad that is tasty.

Soy products

These products are a great protein source plus they have lots of fiber, therefore it is not a surprise that soy is considered to be a staple for the vegetarian's diet. These products come in a lot of versatile forms while being relatively inexpensive, so it offers a great substitute for meat products. Since it has a GI of 16, it fits well in your diet program. Try adding some tempeh, tofu, or soy-beans into your meals to get a diet that is filling and nutritious.

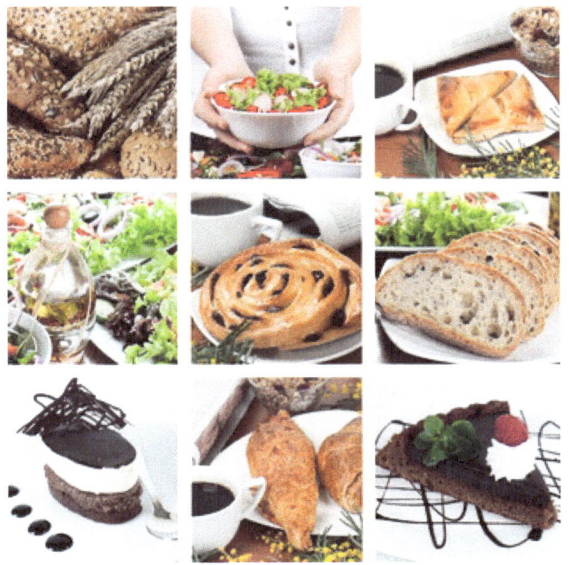

Low-fat Yogurt

Several yogurt brands are found with a GI rating of 16, plus they have ample amount of protein for keeping you feeling full. Yogurt is a healthy pick for breakfast or maybe a snack for any period of the day, plus it can be mixed with a fruit to make a filling, sweet treat. Frozen yogurt also makes a wonderful ice cream substitute, so you can indulge without the guilt!

Oats

They make a nice breakfast food, having a GI of only 36, throughout the morning they will keep persons feeling energized. It can be consumed with yogurt, alone as porridge. There are many ways persons can enjoy their oats as a filling and healthy snack or meal.

Plums

These great healthy tasty fruits are a treat, having a GI of just 24. Nutritious and Sweet sliced up or on their own, plums are perfect in a salad or even with some yogurt.

Legumes

Soy-beans, as well as other delicious legumes, have a low GI. These include: lentils with a GI of 16, which has lots of fiber, folate and iron, chickpeas with a GI of 26. Hummus and red kidney beans have a GI rating of 22, which is perfect for putting a Mexican twist in your meals.

Multi-grain bread

Having a GI lower than 42, a great option for your sandwiches is multi-grain bread, as the grains aid in controlling blood sugar levels and slow digestion. Some other great bread includes linseed and soy and sourdough breads, both can have GI's as low as thirty-six.

Apples

Delicious, crunchy and refreshing apples are a healthy great snack that individuals can eat any time and carry with them anywhere. Apples GI can be as low as twenty-eight, giving them the title as one of the most common consumed low GI fruits. They can be had whole or cut up and added to a salad. There are lots of versatile ways to enjoy apples and it has many healthy advantages.

Most Vegetables

Stock up on greens. The majority of vegetables really are low GI; this means veggies are a great method for adding volume to meals. Here are several top low GI veggies, these include: onions (10), capsicum (10), chilis (10), lettuce (10), cabbage (10), mushrooms (10), broccoli (10), tomatoes (15), cauliflower (15), eggplant (15), carrots (16), frozen corn (47), frozen peas (39).

Chapter 4 - More PCOS Recipes

Curry Chicken

A beautifully flavored curry, prepared with red lentils and chicken. This low GI, low fat, curry is simple to prepare and stay true to an Indian taste. Overall, the glycemic index is lowered by the chicken and the lentils, both ingredients have a low GI index. It is a mouthwatering healthy meal that can be enjoyed at anytime.

<u>Suggested Nutritional Information: remember rice is not included per serving</u>.

Protein: 35g, Calories: 345, Fat: 5g (Cholesterol: 54mg, Saturated: 1g), Sodium: 650mg, Fiber: 17g, Carbohydrate: 37g (Sugars: 4g).

Ingredients

For 4 Servings

3 chicken breasts (medium sized)

200g/7oz red split lentils

2 small onions or 1 large

Optional: ½ green fresh chilli

Ground turmeric (1 tea spoon)

Curry (2 teaspoon of your preferred powder)

Freshly chopped ginger (1 teaspoon)

Salt (1 teaspoon)

Whole cumin seeds (1 teaspoon)

Garlic (3 cloves)

Cayenne pepper (½ teaspoon)

Lemon juice (2 tablespoons)

Ground cinnamon (¼ teaspoon)

Ground nutmeg (¼ teaspoon)

Peel then chop finely 1/2 of the ginger and place it in a pot with the curry powder, turmeric, lentils and sliced onions. If you prefer your curries hot go ahead and add the green sliced chilli.

Add to the pan 1 liter (2 pints) of water then cover using a lid and allow it to simmer for forty minutes. The heat should be low. Leave lid slightly ajar to prevent the contents from boiling over.

Before placing in pot, cut chicken into small cubes then cook for an additional twenty-five minutes until the meat is cooked through. It is crucial for you to remember to regularly stir the pot (every five-ten minutes) to prevent food from burning.

Heat oil in a frying pan then fry the cumin seeds for thirty seconds. Place the remaining garlic and chopped ginger in pan and fry for an additional minute. Cayenne pepper can now be added to the pot, mixed with all the other spices and immediately added to the main pot. Add the cinnamon, nutmeg, salt and lemon juice inside the main pan and for an additional 3 minutes let it cook. Serve with basmati or long grain rice.

Variations

If you prefer your curry fruity then chopped apricots (a handful) can be added at the same time the chicken is added.

Apricot Spiced Turkey

A spicy and tender moist turkey breast including dried apricots gives a nice fruity flavor.

Per serving suggested nutritional information

Sodium: 403mg, Fiber: 4g, Fat: 3g (Cholesterol: 81mg, Saturated: 1g), Protein: 36g, Calories: 323, Carbohydrate: 42g (34g: sugars)

Ingredients

For serving four

Turkey breasts (4)

Rind of one thinly shredded orange

225g /8oz of dried apricots

1 cup /9oz /250g unsweetened yogurt

Ground cumin (1 table spoon)

Ground turmeric (2 tea spoon)

Ground coriander (2 tea spoon)

2 cloves of crushed garlic

Pepper

2 pinches of salt

Horizontally cut every turkey breast down the center; this will make 2 thin slices. Put some pepper and orange rind to one side of all the slices; then place the dried apricots on top.

Turkey slices should be rolled so they can be wrapped around the apricots then a cocktail stick inserted to keep the roll together.

The yogurt is then to be mixed with the garlic, pepper, salt, turmeric cumin, and coriander. Rub or brush the sauce on the rolled turkey breasts.

Add the turkey to a dish then cook in an oven preheated to Gas Mark 5/380°F/190°C for 30 to 35 minutes. After check if the turkey is cooked properly. Serve with broccoli and long-grain white rice.

Beef Stew in Red Wine

This warming stew with red wine is excellent for cold winter days.

Per serving suggested nutritional information

Protein: 26g, Calories: 365, Fat: 6g (Cholesterol: 37mg, Saturated: 2g)

Carbohydrate: 15g (6g Sugars), Sodium: 504mg, Fiber: 3g

Ingredients

(Serves four)

Lean beef (450g)

Carrots (4)

Celery (7 sticks)

Garlic (5 cloves)

Red wine (½ bottle)

Balsamic vinegar (2 tablespoons)

Handful of fresh basil

1 stock cube

Pepper and ground salt

Peel the carrots then chop the celery into chunks approximately ¾ inch thick. Next remove the garlic skin and finely slice, then chop the beef in chunks about ¾ inch thick removing all visible fat.

At high temperature heat sunflower oil (a tablespoon) then braise the exterior of the beef for thirty seconds. Then add the celery, carrot and garlic, and cook for an additional minute.

Finally, add the pepper, salt, basil, vinegar and wine and dissolve or crumble the stock cube in the pan. After lowering heat cover the pot and let stew cook for 1½ to 2 hours. Serve with sourdough bread or pita.

About The Author

PCOS is the abbreviation for Polycystic Ovarian Syndrome which is described as a disorder of the hormones. It is known as a hormonal disorder, which is exceptionally common among women and affects about 7% of them in the world population.

Chantelle Williams is among this estimated percentage. Her first instinct, after being told that it was a possibility that she had PCOS, was to panic because her knowledge of the symptoms that typically comes with it. These are physically and emotionally draining. She started experiencing the heartbreaking symptoms soon after her second of three children.

After her initial shock, Chantelle went into research mode where she set out to find out all she could about the disorder and how to most effectively deal with it. She writes this book for women like herself who might be having the symptoms, but not sure what the cause might be.

The symptoms of this disorder are usually different from one woman to the next, but she advises women who are experiencing obesity, absent or irregular periods, acne, infertility, lipid abnormalities, among other things, to visit their doctor and discuss the symptoms with him or her. Also, she would like viewers to be aware that a visit to the doctor will not confirm PCOS; there has to be blood testing of several different hormones.

www.ingramcontent.com/pod-product-compliance
Lightning Source LLC
Chambersburg PA
CBHW050846290526
45792CB00002B/539